T0156347

BASIC HEALTH
PUBLICATIONS
USER'S GUIDE

TO
ST. JOHN'S
WORT

*Don't Be a Dummy.
Become an Expert on
What St. John's Wort
Can Do for Your
Health.*

LAUREL VUKOVIC
JACK CHALLEM Series Editor

The information contained in this book is based upon the research and personal and professional experiences of the author. It is not intended as a substitute for consulting with your physician or other health care provider. Any attempt to diagnose and treat an illness should be done under the direction of a health care professional.

The publisher does not advocate the use of any particular health care protocol but believes the information in this book should be available to the public. The publisher and author are not responsible for any adverse effects or consequences resulting from the use of the suggestions, preparations, or procedures discussed in this book. Should the reader have any questions concerning the appropriateness of any procedures or preparation mentioned, the author and the publisher strongly suggest consulting a professional health care advisor.

Series Editor: Jack Challem
Editor: Carol Rosenberg
Typesetter: Gary A. Rosenberg
Series Cover Designer: Mike Stromberg

Basic Health Publications User's Guides are published by Basic Health Publications, Inc.

CONTENTS

INTRODUCTION

Everyone suffers from passing moods. True, it doesn't feel good to be sad, blue, or down-in-the-dumps, but changing emotions are a part of what makes us human. It's not realistic to expect to always be happy, or to always feel good. Feelings of sadness and loss are a normal part of life.

However, severe or persistent feelings of sadness or hopelessness erode well-being and significantly interfere with the enjoyment of daily life and the ability to function normally. According to the World Health Organization, major depression is the leading cause of disability in the United States and throughout the rest of the world. The National Institute of Mental Health reports the sobering fact that approximately 17 million American adults suffer from depression each year—more than are stricken with cancer or heart disease.

Fortunately, depressive disorders are highly treatable illnesses. Great strides have been made in recent decades in the physiological and psychological treatment of depression, including natural approaches to treating depressive disorders. By reading this book, you'll gain an understanding of depression and the many things that you can do to alleviate these debilitating conditions.

In *User's Guide to St. John's Wort*, you'll learn about depression and who it affects. You'll find clear descriptions of the symptoms of depressive disorders, along with a simple self-test for depression. Most important, you will learn a great deal of information about effective treatments for depressive disorders. You'll discover the pros and cons of the prescription drugs that are so commonly prescribed for treating depression, and you'll gain a solid knowledge of the natural alternatives available. You'll understand why one of the most highly regarded, well-researched, effective, and safe alternatives to prescription antidepressants is the herb St. John's wort.

In this book, you'll find in-depth and simple-to-understand answers to your questions about St. John's wort. You'll find out how to safely use St. John's wort, and you'll be informed about the most effective forms and dosages of this herb. There are many scientific studies that support the use of this valuable herb for the treatment of depression, and you'll learn about some of these important studies in these pages.

First things first. Read on to discover more about exactly what St. John's wort is, and how it has come to be a renowned herbal treatment for depression.

CHAPTER 1

So You're
Curious about
St. John's Wort

If you're reading this book, you've most likely heard something about St. John's wort. You've probably heard that it can help alleviate feelings of depression. And you might be wondering if St. John's wort could be helpful for you or someone you know.

Perhaps you've been feeling blue lately or have struggled with depression for a long time. Or you might be feeling anxious and are having difficulty sleeping. You might even have tried antidepressant medications, but are unhappy with the side effects or would like to try a more natural approach.

If you are suffering from depression, St. John's wort, an herb with a long history of use in the treatment of emotional distress, may be helpful for you. In a nutshell, it has been found to be most beneficial for people suffering from mild to moderate depression. It's also been found to be helpful for alleviating anxiety and insomnia related to depression, and for depression related to premenstrual syndrome (PMS), menopause, and seasonal affective disorder (SAD).

What Is St. John's Wort?

A perennial plant native to Europe, St. John's wort (*Hypericum perforatum*) has naturalized and grows abundantly along roadsides and other sunny open spaces throughout North and South America, Asia,

Africa, and Australia. It was most likely introduced to North America by early European colonists, and is now grown commercially because of its valuable medicinal properties.

St. John's wort is a nondescript, weedy looking plant that is easy to overlook until mid-summer, when it bursts into a flush of tiny, bright yellow star-shaped flowers. The small, oval leaves are dotted with tiny perforations, hence the species name, *perforatum.*

Hypericin
A natural chemical compound found in St. John's wort that is considered to be one of the herb's primary active ingredients.

If you crush a fresh flower bud, it will release a deep reddish purple oil. This substance is called hypericin, and is considered to be one of the primary active ingredients that gives St. John's wort its healing properties.

One theory as to the origin of the common name of the herb is that early Christians named St. John's wort in honor of John the Baptist. The plant blooms around the time of St. John's Day (June 24) and the herb was traditionally collected on this day, steeped in olive oil to release its blood-red color, and used as an anointing oil to symbolize the blood of the saint. The Latin botanical name *Hypericum* is derived from the Greek word *yper,* which means "upper," and the word *eikon,* which means "image." Early Greeks and Romans placed St. John's wort in their homes above statues of their gods as a protection against evil spirits.

Historical Uses of St. John's Wort

In ancient Europe, St. John's wort was believed to have protective powers against the unseen forces of evil. In Greece and Rome, the herb was used for protection against sorcerer's spells, and early Christians believed that St. John's wort drove away evil spirits. It may be that the people who were considered to be possessed by evil spirits were actually suffering from mental illness and were helped by using St. John's wort. By the time the colonists brought St. John's wort to America, the herb had a reputation for being effective as an antidepressant and for topical wound healing.

Throughout more than 2,000 years of use as a healing herb, St. John's wort has been valued for treating nerve injuries, inflammation, sciatica, ulcers, and burns. But the most compelling use that has brought St. John's wort to the forefront of herbal medicine and the attention of millions of people was the confirmation of the herb's remarkable effects as a natural antidepressant.

Since 1979, St. John's wort has been the subject of more than two dozen rigorous, double-blind, controlled clinical studies. Most of these studies were conducted in Europe, which has a long history of using herbs as alternatives to drugs in the treatment of mental and physical diseases. These well-designed studies have shown that St. John's wort is just as effective as pharmaceutical drugs for treating mild to moderate depression. As a result, St. John's wort is one of the most prescribed treatments for mild to moderate cases of depression in Germany, and has become one of the top ten best-selling dietary supplements in the United States. In 1998, United States consumers purchased $170 million dollars worth of St. John's wort.

St. John's Wort—A Hidden Healer

Although St. John's wort was known as a valuable healing herb for thousands of years, it's only been within the past few years that the herb's value has been fully recognized in the United States. That's because herbal medicine, along with other forms of healing like homeopathy that are now considered "alternative medicine," were edged out of popular use by the rise of the conventional medical establishment many decades ago.

From the mid-1800s through the 1930s, there were two primary schools of medicine practiced in the United States. The orthodox physicians (known as "regulars") practiced conventional medicine, while the Eclectic physicians relied heavily on the use of herbs for healing, much as naturopathic physicians do today. With the discovery of pharmaceutical antibiotics, which appeared to work miracles, orthodox medicine gained a position of power in the United States and drove out the Eclectics.

Naturopathy
A method of treating illness that relies on herbs, diet, and other natural approaches to restore the body to health.

But as we've seen in recent decades, so-called miracle drugs can be a double-edged sword. The antibiotics that were hailed as cures for contagious and often deadly diseases did, in fact, cure individuals. But the overuse and overprescribing of those drugs have created strains of even deadlier antibiotic-resistant bacteria. Epidemiologists and scientists warn that these bacteria could cause mass epidemics, which essentially puts us back at square one in the fight against contagious disease.

The same thing is happening with the medical establishment's reliance on antidepressant drugs. These drugs, especially the most recent varieties, have been prescribed as mood-enhancers for millions of Americans. Touted as safe and effective, three antidepressant medications (Prozac, Zoloft, and Paxil) are among the top-ten selling prescription medications in the United States. But the backlash of overprescribing antidepressants is now being recognized, as more and more stories about unpleasant and lethal side effects—including suicide—and the difficulties of withdrawing from these drugs are coming to light.

How St. John's Wort Gained Recognition

Fortunately, herbal medicine never took a beating in Europe the way it did in the United States. European doctors have always regarded herbs as legitimate medical treatments, and herbal products are commonly sold in European pharmacies. The consumer-driven trend toward natural medicine, including herbal medicine, has fueled the popularity of herbs, including St. John's wort. The long history of St. John's wort as a safe and effective treatment for depression and the dozens of well-researched studies that provide scientific support for St. John's wort make it a logical choice as a natural remedy for alleviating mild to moderate depression.

St. John's wort is the most thoroughly researched of all natural antidepressant remedies. It has been shown to relieve the sadness, irritability, anxiety, hopelessness, sleep disturbances, exhaustion, and other symptoms of depression as well as prescription antidepressants. There are several advantages to using St. John's wort instead of pharmaceutical drugs: St. John's wort has far fewer side effects than drugs (and when side effects do occur, they tend to be minor), St. John's wort extracts cost significantly less than pharmaceutical antidepressants, and patients tend to report greater satisfaction with St. John's wort than with drugs.

Today, St. John's wort is approved by the German Commission E, a regulatory agency similar to the U.S. Food and Drug Administration (FDA), for internal use for the treatment of depression and anxiety, and externally for the treatment of wounds, burns, bruises, and muscle pain.

CHAPTER 2

UNDERSTANDING AND DIAGNOSING DEPRESSION

Occasional feelings of sadness in response to life situations and disappointments are a normal part of being human. Losing a job, moving and leaving behind friends, relationship difficulties, children leaving home, a serious or chronic illness, or the death of a loved one all can bring on feelings of sadness and loss. However, these passing states, although commonly labeled as depression, are very different from the serious illness known as a depressive disorder.

Sadness versus Depression

Distinguishing between normal feelings of sadness and clinical depression is an important first step in recognizing and treating a depressive disorder. It can be a challenging task, because the fluctuating moods that are typical of everyday life can make differentiating between normal and abnormal challenging. Psychiatrists and psychotherapists diagnose someone as being clinically depressed if the person has had at least five specific symptoms of depression for at least two weeks, or if the symptoms have significantly impaired the person's ability to function at work, at school, or in relationships. (In the next chapter, you'll find out more about these specific symptoms.)

Although we tend to think of depression as involving the mind, it also has a significant effect on

SYMPTOMS OF DEPRESSION

- Prolonged sadness or unexplained crying spells.

- Significant changes in appetite or sleep patterns.

- Irritability, anger, worry, agitation, anxiety.

- Pessimism, indifference.

- Loss of energy, persistent tiredness.

- Feelings of guilt, worthlessness.

- Inability to concentrate, indecisiveness.

- Inability to take pleasure in former interests.

- Unexplained aches or pains.

- Recurring thoughts of death or suicide.

the body. Depression impairs well-being on many levels, and interferes with normal patterns of sleeping, eating, exercise, work, relationships, and leisure. Depression significantly affects thoughts, moods, and behaviors. It's not uncommon for a person who is depressed to lose interest in life, even to the point of thinking about suicide.

It's important to realize that anyone can suffer from depression. Certainly, depression is not a sign of weakness, nor is it something of which to be ashamed. In fact, some very prominent people in history—including Abraham Lincoln, Ludwig von Beethoven, Mark Twain, Georgia O'Keefe, and Vincent Van Gogh—have suffered from depression. No one is guaranteed immunity—people of every age, religion, race, and economic and social group are stricken with depression.

Fortunately, through medical research and

modern psychotherapy, we have learned a great deal about depression and how to effectively treat it. According to the American Psychiatric Association, up to 90 percent of all cases of depression can be treated. But it's essential to recognize the need for help. The National Institute of Mental Health reports that two of every three people who suffer from depression don't get the help they need.

Some people simply aren't aware that they are suffering from a depressive disorder. They know that they aren't feeling well, but may think that their symptoms are caused by fatigue or stress. Others are too ashamed to seek help, or may be so worn down by their depression that making the effort to get help is too overwhelming to consider. And according to the National Alliance for the Mentally Ill, professionals may even have a difficult time making a clear diagnosis of a depressive disorder. They report that, on average, it takes almost eight years from the onset of depression for an individual to obtain a proper diagnosis.

The Different Faces of Depression

The most common types of depression are major depression, dysthymia, and bipolar disorder. Major depression (also known as unipolar depression) tends to occur in episodes, and can be so debilitating that it becomes difficult for the sufferer to perform the basic tasks of daily life, or even to get out of bed. This severe form of depression tends to be a chronic, recurring illness.

Major Depression
A form of depression that tends to occur in episodes; so debilitating that it becomes difficult for the sufferer to per - form the basic tasks of daily life.

Although a traumatic life event can provoke a major depressive episode, not all stressful events cause depression, and not all depressive episodes are triggered by a stressful event. According to the U.S. Department of Health and Human Services, major depression affects approximately 15 percent of Americans at some time in life. In economic terms, depression costs the United States approximately $43 billion a year in lost productivity, absenteeism, and medical costs, estimates the National Depressive and Manic Depressive Association. The costs to a human life are immeasurable. Tragically, approximately 15 percent of those who suffer from chronic depression will eventually commit suicide.

Symptoms of depression include persistent feelings of sadness, crying spells, feelings of hopelessness, a loss of pleasure in activities that previously were enjoyed, significant changes in appetite or body weight, difficulty sleeping or sleeping excessively, decreased energy, loss of sexual desire, difficulty concentrating or making decisions, restlessness and irritability, feelings of worthlessness or guilt, and thoughts of death or suicide. Recurring physical symptoms such as headaches, chronic pain, and chronic digestive disorders can also be part of the profile of depression. A person is diagnosed with major depression (also called major depressive disorder or unipolar major depression) if they have five or more of these symptoms persisting for two weeks or longer.

Dysthymia
A milder form of depression with chronic symptoms that can persist for years.

Dysthymia is a less severe form of depression that takes the form of chronic symptoms that can persist for years. People with dysthymia often suffer from low energy, fatigue, sleep disturbances (either oversleeping or insomnia), and appetite disturbances (either poor appetite or overeating).

An individual suffering from dysthymia can generally go about the business of attending to the necessities of daily life, but she feels a persistent lack of pleasure or joy, does not function at her best, and may frequently be irritable and complain of stress. Because they are able to function in daily life, many people with dysthymia are unaware that they are suffering from a depressive disorder. As a result, they don't seek help, but endure the symptoms of depression and the subsequent loss of pleasure and productivity that characterize a healthy life.

Approximately 10 million Americans suffer from dysthymia each year. A diagnosis of dysthymia is made when a depressed mood in an adult persists for at least two years (one year in children or adolescents) and the mood is accompanied by at least two other symptoms of depression.

Bipolar disorder, more commonly known as manic-depressive illness, is less common than the other types of depression, and affects only about one percent of Americans. There is often a family history of manic depression in people who develop this illness. Bipolar disorder usually strikes in late adolescence, often first appearing as depression. But it can also develop in early childhood, or the initial episode may occur in mid-life.

Bipolar disorder is characterized by episodes of major depression that alternate with excessively elevated moods known as mania. Symptoms of mania include irritability, excessive talking, a decreased need for sleep, racing thoughts, agitation, overly inflated self-esteem, inappropriate social behavior, and impulsive behaviors that may involve dangerous activities.

The depressive symptoms of bipolar disorder parallel those of major (unipolar) depression. Because of this, and the fact that manic episodes don't often make an appearance until a person reaches their mid-twenties, people with bipolar disorder may be diagnosed simply with depression. This can be problematic, because the use of antidepressants can bring on a manic episode in someone who actually has bipolar disorder. Working closely with a mental health professional who is skilled in the treatment of bipolar disorder is essential.

Although the mood shifts between depression and mania can be sudden, they most often take place gradually over a period of weeks or months. Many people who have bipolar disorder notice that they tend to feel depressed more often in the winter and have symptoms of mania more frequently in the spring.

Bipolar Disorder
A depressive disorder characterized by episodes of major depression that alternate with excessively elevated moods known as mania.

It's important to note that depression varies from person to person, and that not everyone who is depressed experiences every symptom. Other variables in depression include the severity of symptoms and the response of the individual to treatment. In the vast majority of cases, however, depression is treatable.

What Causes Depression?

Depression has many different causes, and researchers and mental health professionals are still attempting to understand this complex disorder. Many studies indicate a biochemical and genetic basis for some types of depression. That's why depression sometimes appears to run in families, with depression recurring through the generations. Studies of identical twins support the theory that depression has a genetic basis. Researchers have found that if one twin suffers from depression, the other has a 70 percent chance of also being depressed (this holds true even if the twins are separated at birth and raised apart from each other).

But not everyone who has a family history of depression will necessarily fall prey to the illness. And many people with no family history of depression become depressed. A variety of other factors, such as a significant loss, or relationship, family, work, school, financial, and social stresses can trigger the onset of depression.

Genetic
A hereditary tendency passed down from one generation to another through the genes.

Coping Styles and Depression

Personality characteristics and coping styles also play a critical role in depression. People with low self-esteem or those who tend to have a pessimistic outlook are more likely to suffer from depression, as are those who have a low tolerance for the stresses of everyday life. A psychological theory of depression developed by Martin Seligman, Ph.D., in the 1960s (known as the "learned helplessness model") demonstrated that animals who were subjected to situations where they were helpless became depressed, and exhibited changes in brain chemistry that were indicative of depression.

When the dogs in his study were given antidepressant drugs, their brain chemistry changed for the better and their depression lifted. However, when the dogs were taught how to gain control over their environment, their brain chemistry also became normal. This study is significant in that it supports the theory that people who feel helpless and hopeless undergo brain chemistry changes that are associated with depression, and that learning to be self-empowered can alleviate depression.

Depression Is Not a Character Flaw

It's important to remember that depression is not a sign of personal weakness, nor is it a character flaw.

Genetics may play a role in personality structure, but for the most part, these behavioral styles are learned at an early age in the individual's family of origin. An emphasis on learning new behavior and thinking patterns is one of the primary psychological approaches to alleviating depression.

Many physicians immediately prescribe drugs to treat depression, but psychotherapy may work just as well, at least in cases of mild to moderate depression. Teaching people to be more optimistic is one of the most powerful techniques for shifting brain chemistry into a healthy balance. In his studies, Seligman observed that optimistic people rarely, if ever, became helpless and depressed. On the other hand, people who had a pessimistic view of life were highly likely to sink into depression when they encountered challenging life stressors.

Behavioral and attitude changes also generally take time and practice, and the appropriate use of antidepressant medications can help to ease the immediate symptoms to make psychological work more beneficial. St. John's wort is an excellent alternative to psychiatric medications because the lack of side effects makes it easier for many patients to tolerate.

Physical Causes of Depression

In addition to genetic causes and learned behavioral styles, physical illness can also be at the root of depression. Serious illnesses such as a heart attack, stroke, cancer, and rheumatoid arthritis are commonly accompanied by feelings of depression. For example, according to the U.S. Department of Health and Human Services, a person who has suffered a heart attack has a 40 percent chance of becoming depressed. Changes in body chemistry, such as the hormonal shifts that occur during menopause and pregnancy, also can trigger depression.

It's essential to check for the possibility of an underlying physiological cause for depression. If the physical causes aren't addressed, then any attempt at treating the depression will be less successful. Some of the common underlying physical disorders that can cause or contribute to depression include nutrient deficiencies, hypoglycemia, hormonal imbalances (particularly insufficient thyroid or adrenal hormones), allergies, and drug use (including alcohol, caffeine, and prescription drugs).

Hormonal Aspects of Depression

A number of hormones have a significant influence on mood. Many times, physicians neglect to consider hormone levels as an important factor in the treatment of depression. For example, low thyroid function (also known as hypothyroidism) is frequently overlooked by physicians as a cause of depression. Even minute decreases in thyroid hormones can negatively affect the body and mind. Other symptoms of hypothyroidism include fatigue, skin dryness, constipation, feeling cold, difficulties concentrating, and weight gain. If you suspect that your thyroid might not be functioning up to par, ask your doctor to perform a complete endocrine workup, including testing for thyroid hormones.

Hypothyroidism
A common condition of low thyroid function that can cause depression.

Adrenal hormones also play a critical role in depression. Long-term stress, which is frequently a precipitating factor in depression, affects the hormonal output of the adrenal glands. An increased level of cortisol (a hormone released during times of stress) causes mood changes such as nervousness, insomnia, anxiety, and depression. Living under highly stressful conditions, or not having adequate coping skills, can cause the adrenal glands to continue secreting cortisol even when the stressful events have subsided.

Cortisol
A hormone secreted by the adrenal glands in response to stress; causes mood changes such as anxiety and depression.

The use of alcohol, recreational drugs, and even prescription drugs can bring on a depressive disorder in susceptible people. And depressive disorders are a common factor in other emotionally based illnesses such as eating disorders, substance abuse, and anxiety disorders.

Even the change of seasons, from summer to winter, can bring on a type of depression known as seasonal affective disorder, or SAD. The symptoms generally begin in the fall, as the days grow shorter and daylight decreases, and last until spring. Seasonal affective disorder is characterized by fatigue, oversleeping, overeating, and anxiety. Researchers believe that this depressive disorder is triggered by a decline in natural mood-enhancing brain chemicals and is associated with the decrease in sunlight during the winter.

Seasonal Affective Disorder
A depressive disorder associated with the decrease in sunlight during the winter.

In many cases, the first episode of a depressive disorder is triggered by a combination of situational and psychological stressors as well as a possible genetic predisposition toward depression. Subsequent episodes of depression may occur in response to mild stressors or without any apparent cause.

CHAPTER 3

WHO SUFFERS FROM DEPRESSION?

Anyone can suffer from depression. According to the National Institute of Mental Health, depressive disorders most often first occur between the ages of twenty and fifty, with the average age of onset about forty. But people of any age can suffer from depression. There are certain characteristics that seem to apply to specific groups of people.

Depression in Women

Women are far more likely than men to be depressed. In fact, women are twice as likely as men to suffer from depression, and approximately one of every four women will experience clinical depression at some time during her life. This statistic holds true regardless of racial or ethnic background or economic status. In women, depression often appears as a pervasive feeling of helplessness and hopelessness.

Fluctuating hormones during the menstrual cycle, pregnancy, and menopause play a role in a woman's susceptibility to depression. As many as one in ten mothers experience depression after childbirth. These feelings range from a relatively mild case of the blues to major clinical depression; in many cases, women who suffer major depression postpartum have often had prior episodes of depression, although they may not have been diagnosed or treated.

Postpartum Depression
Depression in women that occurs after childbirth.

Because they feel badly about feeling depressed at a time when they think they should be especially happy, women may have difficulties seeking help. Not surprisingly, many women also find the increased stresses of juggling work, family, and household responsibilities cause anxiety and depression.

Depression in Men

Although men are not diagnosed with depression as often as are women, the incidence of depression in men may be higher than it appears. Men are less likely to acknowledge feeling depressed, and tend to cover up their feelings with excessive alcohol or drug use. Many men also bury their depressed feelings in working long hours.

Because depression in men often takes the form of anger, irritability, and emotional withdrawal, others may not realize that a man is depressed. Even physicians are less likely to suspect depression in a man than in a woman. To complicate matters, although a man may be aware of feeling depressed, he is much less inclined than a woman to seek help. This may be the reason why the rate of suicide in men is four times that of women, despite the fact that more women make suicide attempts.

Depression in Children

It's only recently that depression in children has been recognized as a serious problem. Mental health professionals estimate that as many as one of every thirty-three children and one in eight adolescents suffers from depression. Children manifest depression in various ways that may not look on the surface like a depressive disorder. Young children may feign illness, resist going to school, or be excessively fearful. Older children may get into trouble at school, do poorly in classes, exhibit an overall negative attitude, and have difficulty getting along with others.

Depression in children can be difficult to recognize because children naturally go through various stages that can be trying for the child and the parent. A warning sign that something is awry is if symptoms of fear, school problems, or a negative attitude persist. Other behaviors to be aware of include frequent absences from school, isolation from peers, or reckless behavior.

Depression in the Elderly

As a group, the elderly have perhaps been the most neglected in both the recognition and treatment of depression. Because so many older people suffer from depression, some people mistakenly believe that depression is a normal part of aging. This is not true, although approximately one-sixth of Americans over the age of sixty-five suffer from a depressive disorder. Because the symptoms may primarily manifest under the guise of fatigue or other physical complaints, depression is often overlooked in the elderly.

For many older people, depression takes the form of a loss of interest in activities that were formerly pleasurable, a sense of hopelessness about the future, and persistent feelings of sadness. Depression is often triggered by the loss of a spouse or chronic health problems. In the elderly, a depressive disorder has the potential for the most serious health consequences. Those who do not receive treatment for depression are more likely to have poor outcomes associated with the treatment of other illnesses such as heart disease and diabetes. In addition, untreated depression is the primary cause of suicide in the elderly.

Depression Is Treatable

A depressive disorder is a serious illness, and it's not likely to go away without some type of treatment. Depression affects the body, mind, and spirit, and permeates all aspects of an individual's life. Without treatment, depression can linger for years, and cause severe suffering for the individual and those who care about him.

Unfortunately, many people who are depressed do not seek help. Many people are not aware that depression is treatable, or they may feel uncomfortable admitting to feelings of depression. It's important to realize that depression is not a sign of weakness, nor is it a passing mood. A person who is depressed cannot simply pull himself together and shake off depression. With appropriate treatment, however, most people who suffer from depression can be helped. The next chapter will help you determine if you, or someone you know, is suffering from depression.

Helping Someone Who Is Depressed

Many times, people who are depressed do not realize that they are suffering from a depressive disorder. If you suspect that someone you care about is depressed, the most important thing you can do is to help her receive appropriate treatment. Encourage her to seek help, and be willing to take the initiative to make and even to take her to appointments.

Offering emotional support is essential. Try to engage the person in conversation, and pay attention to what she is saying. However, don't try to act as a therapist, and resist the urge to try to solve her problems. Instead, just listen and give the person an opportunity to share her feelings. As trying as it can be to relate to a depressed person, be as patient as possible and remember that someone suffering from a depressive disorder cannot just "snap out" of her depression.

A depressed person needs to know that he has the loving support of his family and friends. Offer encouragement and try to engage the depressed person in simple activities such as a walk or going to a movie. Even if he resists, be persistent in a supportive, gentle, and encouraging manner. Don't be too pushy, because if the person feels like he cannot live up to your expectations or demands, he will feel like a failure and may become more depressed. Remember—and remind the depressed person—that with time and appropriate treatment, he will begin to feel better.

If at any time a depressed person talks about suicide, report this to his therapist. If you suspect that the person may be planning a suicide attempt, call 911 and his therapist right away.

CHAPTER 4

ARE YOU DEPRESSED?
A SIMPLE SELF-TEST

If you suspect depression in yourself or in someone you know, this simple self-test can serve as a gauge to help you decide whether or not to seek professional help. There are no right or wrong answers to this test. The more truthful you can be, the more accurately you can determine your emotional state.

Please note that this test is not a substitute for a therapeutic evaluation. Only a properly trained health professional can accurately diagnose whether or not you are suffering from a depressive disorder. But answering these questions can help you sort through your feelings and communicate your symptoms to your doctor or therapist.

Answer the following questions about how you have been feeling during the past two weeks.

Self-Test for Depression

1. I've been feeling sad or unhappy.

_____ Never or rarely   _____ Sometimes

_____ Often   _____ Most of the time

2. I feel tired and don't have much energy.

_____ Never or rarely   _____ Sometimes

_____ Often   _____ Most of the time

3. I'm sleeping more than usual (or less than usual).

_____ Never or rarely   _____ Sometimes
_____ Often   _____ Most of the time

4. My sleep is restless and disturbed.

_____ Never or rarely   _____ Sometimes
_____ Often   _____ Most of the time

5. I'm eating more than usual (or less than usual).

_____ Never or rarely   _____ Sometimes
_____ Often   _____ Most of the time

6. I feel restless and irritable.

_____ Never or rarely   _____ Sometimes
_____ Often   _____ Most of the time

7. I find it difficult to concentrate or to think clearly.

_____ Never or rarely   _____ Sometimes
_____ Often   _____ Most of the time

8. I don't enjoy activities that I used to find pleasurable.

_____ Never or rarely   _____ Sometimes
_____ Often   _____ Most of the time

9. I'm not interested in sex, or I'm having sexual difficulties.

_____ Never or rarely   _____ Sometimes

_____ Often   _____ Most of the time

10. I have headaches or other pains and my doctor can't find a cause.

_____ Never or rarely   _____ Sometimes

_____ Often   _____ Most of the time

11. I feel as though no one really likes me.

_____ Never or rarely   _____ Sometimes

_____ Often   _____ Most of the time

12. I feel unattractive.

_____ Never or rarely   _____ Sometimes

_____ Often   _____ Most of the time

13. I feel guilty without any real reason.

_____ Never or rarely   _____ Sometimes

_____ Often   _____ Most of the time

14. I feel fearful and anxious.

_____ Never or rarely   _____ Sometimes

_____ Often   _____ Most of the time

15. I have negative, critical thoughts about myself.

_____ Never or rarely   _____ Sometimes

_____ Often   _____ Most of the time

16. I feel hopeless.

_____ Never or rarely   _____ Sometimes

_____ Often   _____ Most of the time

17. I feel like a failure in life.

_____ Never or rarely   _____ Sometimes

_____ Often   _____ Most of the time

18. My life feels empty and nothing seems worth doing.

_____ Never or rarely   _____ Sometimes

_____ Often   _____ Most of the time

19. I don't feel like I will ever feel better.

_____ Never or rarely   _____ Sometimes

_____ Often   _____ Most of the time

20. I have thoughts of death or suicide.

_____ Never or rarely   _____ Sometimes

_____ Often   _____ Most of the time

When you finish taking the test, tally up your responses in each category. Assign each "Never or rarely" answer 1 point; each "Sometimes" answer 2 points; each "Often" answer 3 points; and each "Most of the time" answer 4 points.

If you scored below 30 points, you are probably not depressed. If you scored between 30 and 50, you are likely mildly or moderately depressed, and should consult a therapist or your doctor for guidance. If you scored over 50 points, you may be suffering from serious depression, and should consult your doctor for help without delay. Preferably, consult a doctor who is open to treating depression in a holistic way.

CHAPTER 5

CONVENTIONAL
TREATMENTS
FOR DEPRESSION

If you think that you or someone you care about is suffering from depression, the first step is to see a doctor for a thorough examination. It's important to rule out physical conditions that can mimic depression. For example, a lingering viral infection can cause fatigue, lethargy, and other symptoms associated with depression. If your doctor finds no physical reason for your symptoms, the next step is to consult a psychologist, psychiatrist, or psychotherapist who can evaluate your symptoms and make a diagnosis.

Diagnosing Depression

Endogenous Depression
Depression that originates from within without apparent relation to external life events.

During a psychological evaluation, you can expect to be asked about the history of your depression, including the symptoms you are experiencing, when they began, and if you have ever suffered from depression in the past. A thorough evaluation will also include questions about drug and alcohol use, any family history of depressive disorders, and previous treatments you may have received for depression. It's important to distinguish between situational depression, which is related to external events such as the loss of a spouse or other stressful life situ-ations, and endogenous depression, which arises internally and is independent of life stressors.

A variety of different medications and treatments are available for treating depressive disorders. Milder forms of depression often respond well to psychotherapy and the use of antidepressants when necessary. People suffering from moderate to severe depression generally do best with a combination of antidepressant medication and psychotherapy. Antidepressants help to shift brain chemistry to alleviate feelings of depression, and psychotherapy provides the opportunity to learn more effective ways of managing life stressors.

Conventional Medical Treatments

The most common conventional medical treatment for depressive disorders is medication; so commonly are these medications prescribed that more than 28 million Americans take antidepressant drugs or anxiety medications. Scientists generally regard depression as

Neurotransmitters *Chemical messengers responsible for transmitting information between nerve cells.*

caused by disordered brain chemistry, and a number of studies support the view that depressed people have imbalances in neurotransmitters, the chemicals in the brain that facilitate communication between nerve cells.

Two neurotransmitters that are thought to be especially important are serotonin and norepinephrine. Both of these brain chemicals are generally found in short supply in people who are depressed. Serotonin is often referred to as the brain's natural mood-elevating drug. It also has relaxing and sedative properties. People who have high levels of serotonin tend to be optimistic, calm, patient, and good natured. They also tend to be focused, creative, and have a good ability to concentrate. Physiologically, they usually sleep well, and do not have an undue craving for carbohydrates.

On the other hand, people with low serotonin levels tend to be depressed, anxious, irritable, and impatient. They typically crave sweets and high-carbohydrate foods, and often suffer from insomnia. The lowest levels of serotonin are found in people who have attempted suicide.

Scientists believe that some people are genetically programmed to produce less serotonin, which can predispose them to depression. But not everyone with this genetic tendency will become depressed, and there are plenty of people who produce sufficient levels of serotonin who are depressed. Clearly, although serotonin plays an important role in depression, there are many other factors involved in the disorder.

Medications for Depression

The U.S. Food and Drug Administration has approved dozens of medications for treating depressive disorders. The medications are classified according to their effects on the various chemicals in the brain. The older antidepressants, first prescribed in the 1950s, include tricyclic antidepressants such as Tofranil (imipramine) and monoamine oxidase inhibitors (MAOIs) such as Nardil (phenelzine). Newer antidepressants, known as selective serotonin reuptake inhibitors (SSRIs), include Prozac (fluoxetine), Zoloft (sertraline), Paxil (paroxetine), Wellbutrin (bupropion), Effexor (venlafaxine), Remeron (mirtazapine), and Serzone (nefazodone). These newer drugs work by increasing serotonin levels.

Understanding how serotonin works in the body helps in understanding something about how these drugs work. Serotonin is manufactured naturally in the brain, and then is stored in nerve cells until it is needed. The job of serotonin is to carry messages to nerve cells. When serotonin is released, it transmits a chemical message to a nerve cell by attaching to a receptor site on the nerve cell. At the same time that serotonin is being released, enzymes in the body go to work either to break down the serotonin or to help it be taken back into the brain cells. Both of these processes reduce the effect of serotonin in the body. The drugs developed to alleviate depression work by either preventing the breakdown of serotonin or inhibiting the reuptake of serotonin into the brain. This means that there is more serotonin available in the body to produce a natural mood-enhancing effect.

While these drugs have demonstrated effectiveness for treating depression, they may not be necessary for mild or moderate cases of depression. There are a number of effective alternatives to antidepressant drugs, including diet and lifestyle changes that help to naturally increase serotonin levels. These factors include balancing blood sugar levels, eating a diet rich in foods that support nervous system health, and regular exercise. You can read more about this in Chapter 8.

In addition, addressing the underlying psychological causes for depression and learning new and more positive ways of coping with life stressors also helps to increase serotonin levels naturally. Chapter 9 goes into detail about the many ways that you can help yourself overcome depressive disorders.

Lifestyle changes and psychotherapy approaches are not magic wands, however. They take time and consistent effort, and results generally do not occur overnight. In the meantime, St. John's wort offers a natural, safe, and effective alternative to antidepressant drugs for providing a boost of serotonin, which helps to ease the symptoms of depression and supports the effort necessary for making life changes.

How Antidepressants Work

Researchers aren't exactly sure how antidepressants work, but they do know that these drugs help to restore chemical balance in the brain, which in turn, helps to alleviate depressive symptoms. For most patients, it takes between four to eight weeks for the drug to fully take effect. To avoid a relapse, many patients remain on antidepressants for six months to one year following a major depressive episode.

No one treatment works best for everyone, and discovering the most effective treatment involves working closely with a doctor who can adjust medications or combinations of medications as needed. Physicians often try a variety of antidepressant medications to find the most effective medication or combination of medications. In general, it takes anywhere from one to two months to obtain the full therapeutic benefit of the drug.

Antidepressants are usually prescribed for at least four months, and in the case of a chronic major depressive disorder or bipolar disorder, medication may need to be taken indefinitely to prevent a recurrence of symptoms. Antidepressants should never be discontinued abruptly; to do so can cause unpleasant withdrawal symptoms.

Although prescription antidepressants can be remarkably effective for treating depression, they are not a cure all nor are they benign substances. For one thing, the drugs don't alleviate depression for everyone. For some people the relief provided by drugs merely softens the edge of depression. It's not unusual for antidepressants to cause side effects. The primary side effects of tricyclic antidepressants are dry mouth, constipation, blurred vision, dizziness, drowsiness, sexual problems, and difficulty urinating. Monoamine oxidase inhibitors (MAOIs) can cause a fatal rise in blood pressure if combined with certain foods or medications. The most common side effects of SSRIs include headache, nausea, agitation, insomnia, and sexual difficulties.

Withdrawal from Antidepressants

One of the most disturbing and least talked about problems with antidepressants is the issue of withdrawal. The brain becomes accustomed to certain levels of serotonin, and some people suffer distress when they either stop taking or take lower doses of serotonin-boosting antidepressants.

In fact, studies indicate that up to 85 percent of patients who take prescription SSRIs have some type of withdrawal symptoms when they stop taking the drug. The symptoms include balance problems, nerve tingling, nausea, flulike symptoms, difficulties sleeping, anxiety, and depression. Many patients continue taking antidepressant drugs unnecessarily because they assume their withdrawal symptoms signify a relapse of depression. Disturbingly, many doctors are not aware that stopping antidepressants can cause such symptoms.

Often, doctors routinely prescribe antidepressants for patients who show any sign whatsoever of depression. In fact, Prozac, which has been on the market since 1988, is the third top-selling drug in the United States. Zoloft, introduced in 1992, is seventh on the list, and Paxil, brought to the market in 1993, is in ninth place. Hailed as the miracle drugs of modern psychiatric medicine, these antidepressants have been prescribed for at least 28 million Americans. But the drawbacks of Prozac and similar antidepressants are now being recognized, just as the problems with Valium and amphetamines (both also used as mood enhancers in the past) came to light a couple of decades ago.

Experts Criticize Antidepressant Drugs

Critics of antidepressant drugs maintain that far too many prescriptions for these drugs are being written. Joseph Glenmullen, M.D., a Harvard psychiatrist and author of *Prozac Backlash*, maintains that the long-term effects of antidepressants have not been considered. He also criticizes the managed health care system in this country for putting people on antidepressants because it's cheaper than paying for psychotherapy. Although he acknowledges that antidepressants can be helpful for people with serious depression, he recommends that people with mild depression should avoid prescription antidepressants, and suggests St. John's wort and psychotherapy as alternative approaches.

Problems arise when people who suffer from mild depression or even those who are simply experiencing an intense period of life stress are started on prescription antidepressants by their doctors, and then suffer withdrawal symptoms when they try to get off of the medication. When they decrease their dosage of the drugs, it can be difficult for the doctor to determine whether the patient's symptoms are caused by withdrawal from the drug, or if the symptoms of the depression are recurring.

The cycle of trying to wean a patient from antidepressants can potentially go on for years, with patients being switched from one drug to another in an attempt to alleviate symptoms. The truth is that very little is known about the long-term effects of modern prescription antidepressants. These drugs were initially approved by the Food and Drug Administration, the government agency responsible for protecting the health of consumers. But once a drug is on the market, the FDA does little in the way of tracking the side effects of long-term use. The FDA itself estimates that only 1 percent to 10 percent of all drug side effects are reported to the agency.

Doctors have the responsibility of informing their patients about the potential adverse effects of antidepressants, as well as how to safely stop taking the drugs. But a report in the *Journal of Clinical Psychiatry* showed that as many as 70 percent of general practitioners and 30 percent of psychiatrists aren't educated about the withdrawal effects of stopping serotonin boosting antidepressants such as Prozac, Zoloft, and Paxil. Of the doctors who are aware, only 17 percent of general practitioners and 20 percent of psychiatrists inform their patients of the correct way to wean themselves from the drugs.

Clearly, as effective as modern antidepressant drugs can be for treating depressive disorders, they are not a panacea, nor do they come without risks. There are, however, a number of alternative approaches to depression that have been shown to be as effective as pharmaceutical drugs, but with few or no side effects. One of the most promising of these alternatives is the herb St. John's wort.

CHAPTER 6

HOW ST. JOHN'S WORT
CAN HELP YOU

Not only is St. John's wort a popular treatment for mild to moderate depression, but it can also be helpful for anxiety, sleep disorders, the mood swings associated with premenstrual syndrome (PMS) and menopause, and seasonal affective disorder (SAD).

A quick recap of depression: People suffering from depressive disorders have an imbalance of specific brain chemicals known as neurotransmitters. This imbalance causes a variety of physical, emotional, and mental symptoms. Physically, these symptoms manifest as changes in sleep, appetite, and energy. Emotionally, the person may feel a sense of hopelessness, irritability, or a lack of interest in work, socializing, or hobbies. And mentally, the person may have difficulties concentrating or making decisions. St. John's wort has proven helpful for alleviating all of these symptoms. As a result, this herb is highly regarded as an alternative to conventional medications for depressive disorders.

St. John's wort plays a prominent role in European herbal medicine, particularly in Germany, where doctors prescribed almost 66 million daily doses of the herb in 1994 for psychological disorders. St. John's wort is clearly the treatment of choice for depressive disorders in Germany—physicians there prescribe extracts of the herb twenty times more often than they do Prozac.

Prescribing St. John's wort as an alternative to pharmaceutical antidepressants makes sense. Pharmaceutical drugs have numerous side effects, including dry mouth, nausea, fatigue, headache, gastrointestinal distress, sleep disturbances, and impaired sexual functioning. In contrast, St. John's wort carries little risk of side effects, and those that are reported, such as gastrointestinal upset, tend to be minor. St. John's wort also costs far less than prescription antidepressants. And St. John's wort does not require a prescription.

If you are currently taking prescription medication for the treatment of a depressive disorder, do not begin taking St. John's wort without consulting with your doctor. The combination of St. John's wort and standard antidepressants can cause side effects. And never discontinue antidepressants without talking with your doctor. While many people have switched from antidepressant drugs to St. John's wort, you should only do so under the supervision of your doctor.

How St. John's Wort Works

Hyperforin
A naturally occurring chemical compound in St. John's wort that has been identified as having anti-depressant effects.

The primary compounds in St. John's wort include flavonoids (hyperoside, quercetin, isoquercitrin, and rutin), hyperforin, hypericin, pseudohypericin, polycyclic phenols, kaempferol, luteolin, and biapigenin. Researchers have not determined which of these compounds are the active ingredients, but there is some consensus that hyperforin has effects on mood. Many St. John's wort products are standardized to contain specific amounts of hypericin and hyperforin, which guarantees that the supplement contains what has been judged by researchers to be a sufficient amount of the herb to have a beneficial effect.

Researchers are still studying St. John's wort to determine exactly how it manages to alleviate depression. Although many clinical studies have proven the effectiveness of St. John's wort in relieving depression, scientists like to have a clear picture of exactly how the herb affects the body and brain. The theories are fairly complex, and it appears that St. John's wort may operate in somewhat roundabout ways to ease depressive symptoms. Some research indicates that St. John's wort acts in a similar way to antidepressive drugs in that it inhibits the rate at which brain cells reabsorb serotonin (the neurotransmitter that aids communication between nerve cells and acts as the body's natural feel-good chemical). People who are depressed often have low levels of serotonin.

Another theory about the beneficial effect of St. John's wort is that it seems to reduce levels of interleukin-6, a protein that plays a role in the communication between cells in the body's immune system. Increased levels of interleukin-6 may stimulate the increase of adrenal regulatory hormones, which are a biological marker for depression. It may be that by reducing interleukin-6, St. John's wort helps to treat depression. More studies are needed (some are currently in progress) to determine precisely what are the active ingredients in St. John's wort, and to figure out exactly how these compounds work. Meanwhile, the following are some of the depressive disorders for which St. John's wort has been found helpful.

St. John's Wort and Anxiety

Anxiety often plays a prominent role in depressive disorders, manifesting as feelings of restlessness, irritability, and insomnia. Other common symptoms of anxiety include muscle tension, digestive upsets, and heart palpitations. A certain level of anxiety is a normal reaction to specific situations—for example, most people feel anxious when faced with a dangerous situation. But constant, chronic anxiety impairs the quality of life and can become debilitating.

Physicians often prescribe benzodiazepine medications such as Valium and Xanax for treating anxiety. These drugs have numerous side effects (including lethargy, drowsiness, and mental impairment) and a high potential for addiction. They can also trigger depression. A much safer alternative is to follow the lifestyle suggestions in this book, making sure to avoid all stimulants such as caffeine. St. John's wort has been found to be as helpful as prescription medications in easing anxiety, but without the harmful side effects.

SAD Relief with St. John's Wort

St. John's wort is not only helpful for chronic depression, but it can also be valuable for treating seasonal affective disorder, also known as SAD. People with this condition are strongly affected by the onset of winter, and suffer from feelings of fatigue, irritability, and depression. The condition is related to the diminishing sunlight that typically occurs during the winter months. Although it's not uncommon to feel the urge to "cocoon" during the winter, people with SAD may become so withdrawn that they find it difficult to perform the normal tasks of daily life. They may also tend to overeat, especially carbohydrates, and spend a greater amount of time sleeping than usual. The symptoms of SAD usually disappear with the return of spring and increasing daylight, but the winter months can become unbearable for those who suffer from the disorder.

One of the most effective treatments for SAD is to spend time every day in full spectrum light, which duplicates the beneficial mood-enhancing properties of sunlight. Light boxes made especially for this purpose are widely available, and symptoms are generally relieved within a week or two of daily exposure. It usually takes at least thirty minutes of daily early morning light therapy for best results. In addition, engaging in regular exercise at midday is helpful for obtaining as much natural light as possible during the winter months.

Prescription antidepressants are often recommended for people suffering from SAD. St. John's wort can be an effective, natural alternative. You may have heard cautions concerning the combination of St. John's wort and sunlight. It's true that St. John's wort can cause photosensitivity (an allergic reaction that occurs with exposure to the ultraviolet rays of sunlight) but it's unlikely to occur in humans. There's absolutely no need to be concerned about the combination of light box therapy and St. John's wort, because light boxes do not produce ultraviolet light.

Photosensitivity
An allergic skin reaction that occurs with exposure to ultraviolet rays.

St. John's Wort and PMS

Premenstrual syndrome (PMS) is one of the most widespread problems afflicting women. By some estimates, as many as 90 percent of women in their reproductive years are affected to some degree by PMS. Mood swings, irritability, insomnia, and depression commonly occur during the week to ten days prior to the onset of menstruation. For some women, PMS symptoms can occur during most of the month.

A study of nineteen women at the University of Exeter in the United Kingdom showed that two-thirds of the women found significant relief when taking St. John's wort. They were given 900 mg (mg) of the herb daily for two complete menstrual cycles, and found that their PMS-related symptoms of depression, anxiety, nervous tension, confusion, and crying were diminished by more than half.

St. John's Wort and Menopause

Menopause is a time of great change on many levels. It's not uncommon for a woman to experience situational depression associated with midlife and the many adjustments that accompany this life transition, such as children leaving home, relationship changes, the loss of youth, and of course, the actual physiological changes of declining hormone levels. Many women find that the perimenopausal and menopausal years bring profound emotions to the surface.

Christiane Northrup, M.D., author of *Women's Bodies, Women's Wisdom,* points out that menopause is often a time when women find themselves facing the "unfinished business" of the first half of their lives. Many women may find that they have spent years denying their real wants and needs, and depression may be a cry from the inner self for acknowledgment. A woman may find that she grieves paths not taken, opportunities missed, and the loss of youth. It's important during this time to not suppress feelings, but to pay attention to them. There is often wisdom and greater self-understanding lying beneath the surface of depression.

Giving yourself the time to fully explore your feelings will help you to free yourself from regrets and to make decisions as to how you want to live the second half of your life. "If a woman is willing to deal with her own unfinished business, she will have fewer menopausal symptoms," says

Northrup. "She will find that her symptoms are messages from her inner guidance system that parts of her life need attention." In addition to self-exploration, dietary improvement, and exercise, Northrup also suggests St. John's wort for supporting a woman who needs extra help alleviating menopausal depression.

Unfortunately, many doctors are too quick to prescribe prescription antidepressants for treating menopausal depression. Lifestyle changes, psychotherapy, and natural remedies present a far safer and healthier alternative. It is much better to avoid drugs, especially in cases of mild to moderate depression, and to use natural therapies combined with appropriate emotional work for healing the underlying psychological distress.

CHAPTER 7

SCIENTIFIC SUPPORT
FOR ST. JOHN'S WORT

The benefits of St. John's wort compared to pharmaceutical prescription drugs have been clearly demonstrated in a number of well-designed clinical studies. A handful of these studies are outlined here to give you an idea of the scientific support for St. John's wort.

Not only has the herb been found to be as effective as prescription drugs such as Prozac and Zoloft, but it also has far less incidence of side effects, and the side effects that do occur, such as dry mouth, tend to be minor. Other studies that you will find mentioned in this chapter include the usefulness of St. John's wort for treating depression in children, and the beneficial effects of St. John's wort on premenstrual depression and menopause in women.

Why Doctors Prescribe Drugs

Unfortunately, even with the numerous studies that demonstrate the effectiveness and safety of St. John's wort for treating mild to moderate depression, many physicians continue instead to prescribe drugs. There are several possible reasons for this. Pharmaceutical companies spend billions of dollars advertising their antidepressant drugs, including ads in the popular media, which influence not only what physicians prescribe, but also what patients request from their doctors. In addition, pharmaceutical companies are generally not interested in researching botanical medicines because they would have difficulties obtaining a patented formula. And the fact that herbal remedies are widely available over the counter in natural food stores and pharmacies significantly limits marketing potential, sales, and income for pharmaceutical manufacturers.

Some physicians also hesitate to prescribe St. John's wort because they aren't accustomed to using herbal remedies. And other doctors may be uncomfortable because all of the precise active ingredients in St. John's wort have not been identified. This is not unusual with botanical medicines. Typically, they contain a wide array of compounds that act in harmony with one another. Trying to isolate one compound and dismissing the rest as unimportant is a short-sighted view that has plagued modern medicine.

As many herbalists and botanical researchers point out, herbs contain a variety of compounds that act synergistically to create a physiological effect in the body, and the complete herb has greater potential for healing than just one isolated chemical constituent. For example, while hyperforin may indeed be the primary active ingredient in St. John's wort that helps to relieve depression, there are other compounds that support the action of hyperforin, and still others that buffer the active ingredients to prevent side effects.

The important point that you will see from the studies below is that St. John's wort is clearly effective for the treatment of mild to moderate depression. It alleviates symptoms, and does so without harm to the patient, which undoubtedly meets anyone's criteria for good medicine.

St. John's Wort versus Placebo

In a study of seventy-two patients comparing St.

John's wort to a placebo, German physicians gave patients either 900 mg of St. John's wort extract or a placebo daily for forty-two days. They found that the patients scores on the Hamilton Depression Scale (a standard test used to measure depression) declined by 55 percent among those taking St. John's wort, and only dropped by 28 percent among those taking the placebo. Those who were given St. John's wort also showed improvement in symptoms after only one week of taking the herb, and showed significant positive response after twenty-eight and forty-two days. The patients reported no side effects.

In addition, an overview of twenty-three clinical trials published in the *British Medical Journal* found that St. John's wort extracts were significantly superior to a placebo in relieving depression, and as effective as standard antidepressants. The studies involved a total of 1,757 outpatients with mild to moderately severe depressive disorders.

St. John's Wort versus Prozac

In a six-week German study, 240 patients suffering from mild to moderate depression were given either 500 mg of St. John's wort daily or Prozac. The patients were assessed using the Hamilton Depression Scale. Both groups showed approximately a 12 percent decline in depressive symptoms at the end of the six weeks.

Patients were also tested using the Clinical Global Impression Scale, which showed that St. John's wort was significantly more effective in relieving depression than Prozac. Only six of the patients taking St. John's wort complained of side effects, and these were gastrointestinal symptoms. But thirty-four of the patients taking Prozac reported side effects, including gastrointestinal problems, vomiting, agitation, dizziness, and erectile dysfunction.

St. John's Wort versus Zoloft

In a seven-week study of thirty depressed patients conducted by Ronald Brenner, M.D., and associates of the St. John's Episcopal Hospital in Far Rockaway, New York, St. John's wort was found to be comparable to Zoloft in relieving depressive symptoms. The patients were given either the prescription antidepressant Zoloft or 600–900 mg of a standardized extract of St. John's wort daily. Depression was measured using the Hamilton Depression Scale and the Clinical Global Impression Scale.

Brenner reported significant improvements in the patients taking St. John's wort within two weeks. Measurements after six weeks showed that depressive symptoms were reduced by an average of 40 percent in patients taking Zoloft, and 47 percent in those taking St. John's wort. Two of the patients taking Zoloft reported symptoms of nausea or headache, and two patients taking St. John's wort reported dizziness.

St. John's Wort versus Tofranil

In two clinical studies, St. John's wort has been shown to be as effective as Tofranil (imipramine), one of the most frequently prescribed tricyclic antidepressants. In a study at the Imerem Institute for Medical Research Management and Biometrics in Nuremberg, Germany, psychiatry professor Michael Philipp, M.D., and his colleagues gave 1,050 mg of St. John's wort extract, Tofranil, or a placebo daily for eight weeks to 263 patients (66 men, 197 women) suffering from moderate depression.

The results, published in the *British Medical Journal*, showed that St. John's wort was superior to the placebo and comparable to Tofranil in relieving the patients' depressive symptoms. Results were measured by the researchers using the Hamilton Anxiety Scale, the Clinical Global Impression Scale, and the Zung Self-Rating Depression Scale. The patients who were given St. John's wort had one-third the incidence of side effects as those taking Tofranil. The chief side effect reported was dry mouth. The researchers noted that St. John's wort is a safe treatment for depression and that it improves quality of life for patients.

St. John's wort also compared well to Tofranil in another German study of 324 patients with mild to moderate depression. Helmut Woelk, M.D., of the University of Giessen, Germany, and his colleagues gave St. John's wort or Tofranil daily to the patients for six weeks. They found that both St. John's wort and Tofranil decreased the symptoms of depression by half. St. John's wort exceeded Tofranil in reducing anxiety, however. The researchers also noted that almost half of the study participants experienced side effects while taking Tofranil, primarily complaining of dry mouth and nausea. In contrast, only 20 percent of the patients taking St. John's wort suffered side effects, most commonly dry mouth.

St. John's Wort and PMS

Many women suffer from depressive symptoms in the week or two prior to menstruation. The Food and Drug Administration has recently approved a form of Prozac, called Serafem, as a treatment for depression associated with premenstrual syndrome. Serafem and St. John's wort have not been directly compared in a clinical study, but St. John's wort has been shown to be an effective treatment for alleviating premenstrual depression.

A study of nineteen women at the University of Exeter in the United Kingdom conducted by Edzard Ernst, M.D., showed that two-thirds of the women found significant relief when taking St. John's wort. They were given 900 mg daily for two complete menstrual cycles, and found that their PMS-related symptoms of depression, anxiety, nervous tension, confusion, and crying were diminished by more than half. No significant side effects were reported by the study participants.

St. John's Wort and Menopause

Depressive symptoms occur frequently in the pre- and postmenopausal years, and cause significant distress for many women. A German study of 111 women found that St. John's wort provides substantial improvement in the psychological and psychosomatic symptoms of menopause.

The women studied were between forty-three and sixty-five years old with symptoms characteristic of the pre- and postmenopausal years. They were given 900 mg of St. John's wort extract (300 mg three times a day) for twelve weeks, and their symptoms were evaluated using the Clinical Global Impression Scale and the Menopause Rating Scale. Symptoms were evaluated after five, eight, and twelve weeks of treatment.

The researchers found that there was significant improvement in menopausal problems, with menopausal complaints diminishing or disappearing completely in the majority of women. The women self-rated their improvement at 76 percent, and their physicians rated the women's improvement at 79 percent. The researchers also noted that the women's sexual well-being was enhanced as a result of treatment with St. John's wort.

St. John's Wort for Childhood Depression

At least one in thirty-three children under the age of twelve suffers from depression, and researchers have found that St. John's wort is as effective and safe for treating childhood depression as it is for adults.

A recent German study by Wolf-Dietrich Huebner, M.D., and Tilman Kirste, M.D., at thirty-five pediatric clinics in Germany evaluated seventy-four children suffering from depressive symptoms, including anxiety, irritability, restlessness, poor concentration, sleep disturbances, feelings of dejection, and lack of motivation. The children, ranging in age from one to twelve, were given 300–1,800 mg of St. John's wort extract daily for four to six weeks.

The study found that 72 percent of the children were "good" or "excellent" responders after only two weeks of taking the herb. After four weeks, the number of positive responses rose to 97 percent, with a full 100 percent evaluated as "good" or "excellent" responders at the end of six weeks. The parents also evaluated their children, and their ratings were almost identical to those of the researchers. While St. John's wort improved most of the children's depressive symptoms, it did not appear to have an affect on their ability to concentrate. There were no side effects noted. However, one child showed an increase in depressive symptoms after starting St. John's wort, but subsequently improved over the following two weeks of taking the herb.

Challenge to St. John's Wort

Last year, a study came out that seemed to dispute the credibility of St. John's wort. The study was published in the *Journal of the American Medical Association,* and the ensuing newspaper headlines reported that St. John's wort had been found useless for the treatment of depression. Unfortunately, this study was very misleading. It was conducted on people suffering from severe depression, for which St. John's wort has never been purported to be the most effective treatment. St. John's wort has been recommended for treating mild to moderate cases of depression, for which it has been found very successful.

It is important to note that this study was funded and organized by Pfizer, the same pharmaceutical company that makes Zoloft, which is one of the most often prescribed conventional antidepressant drugs.

Numerous previous clinical studies have supported the use of St. John's wort for the treatment of depression. These studies have demonstrated that St. John's wort is not only as effective as prescription antidepressants, but it has far fewer and much less severe side effects. And even this controversial study did acknowledge that a few patients, although they suffered from severe depression, did actually benefit from taking St. John's wort.

CHAPTER 8

ALLEVIATE DEPRESSION WITH DIET AND EXERCISE

It's not news that nutrition has a direct effect on your physical well-being, as many studies over the past few decades have proven. Heart disease, high blood pressure, cancer, and diabetes are a few of the many diseases that have been shown to be directly affected by diet. But many people are unaware that food choices also play a significant role in emotional and mental well-being.

Eat Right to Combat Depression

Nutrition affects not only your daily moods, but is also a factor in the onset and progression of depression. Your brain requires an adequate and steady supply of nutrients and quickly shows signs of stress when your diet is inadequate. While people vary somewhat in their dietary needs, the following guidelines are usually helpful for most people who suffer from mood swings and depression.

Keeping blood sugar levels balanced is essential for those who are prone to depression. The brain and nervous system are highly sensitive to blood sugar fluctuations. In addition, keeping blood sugar stable ensures a constant supply of energy for the body, which helps to prevent fatigue. To keep blood sugar levels on an even keel, avoid sugary foods and refined carbohydrates, which are quickly converted to sugar in the body. Obviously, desserts and sweets are usually loaded with sugar, but other foods such as salad dressings and dry cereals often contain large amounts of sweeteners.

Some of the many guises of sugar include sucrose, glucose, maltose, dextrose, and corn syrup. Even sweeteners that are thought to be healthful alternatives, such as honey, maple syrup, barley malt, and molasses have a detrimental effect on blood sugar. Ideally, eat sugar primarily as it occurs in whole foods, such as fresh fruits and sweet vegetables such as carrots, winter squashes, and sweet potatoes, and reserve concentrated sweets for occasional treats. Other foods that interfere with healthy blood sugar levels include refined carbohydrates made from white flour, which are rapidly broken down into simple sugars during digestion.

Also avoid caffeine and alcohol, which cause blood sugar fluctuations and have other negative effects on the body. Caffeine is a powerful stimulant drug that stresses the nervous system and contributes to anxiety, irritability, and insomnia. It overstimulates the adrenal glands, creating a state of chronic stress, and results in fatigue after the initial stimulant effect wears off.

To ensure a constant supply of nutrients that keep blood sugar levels balanced, eat small meals several times a day. Choose from high-complex carbohydrates, lean proteins, and healthful fats. High complex carbohydrates, such as legumes, whole grains, nuts, seeds, vegetables, and fruits provide a steady source of energy for the body and brain. Avoid skipping meals or going for more than three hours without eating. For optimal blood sugar control, eat three moderate meals daily plus a mid-morning, mid-afternoon, and a before-bed snack.

Natural Antidepressant Foods

Keeping blood sugar levels in balance is important

for stabilizing mood and increasing energy and well-being. But don't stop there. The foods you choose to eat on a daily basis can actually have a significant antidepressant effect.

Nerve cells in the brain communicate through chemicals called neurotransmitters, which are dependent upon specific nutrients in the blood. Prescription antidepressants work by increasing levels of neurotransmitters, but you can also increase these mood-elevating substances with foods and nutritional supplements. Protein-rich foods such as chicken, turkey, fish, eggs, lentils, almonds, tofu, and yogurt are made up of amino acids, which are the building blocks for neurotransmitters. To ensure an adequate supply of protein in your diet, eat a small serving of protein at each meal and include a bit of protein (such as a few nuts or a small piece of cheese) with each snack, for a total of approximately 8 to 10 ounces of protein daily.

Essential fatty acids are another important nutrient for alleviating depression. They play a critical role in maintaining healthy cell membranes, which are involved in the synthesis and transmission of neurotransmitters. Depression is associated with low levels of essential fatty acids, particularly omega-3 fatty acids and gamma linolenic acid (GLA). Omega-3 fatty acids are thought to enhance the responsiveness of nerve cells to serotonin, the brain's natural mood-uplifting chemical.

Omega-3 fatty acids are found in cold-water fish such as salmon, mackerel, sardines, trout, and albacore tuna; walnuts; and flaxseeds. To obtain sufficient amounts of omega-3 fatty acids, eat cold-water fish at least three times a week (daily is better if you are suffering from depression), and eat a small handful of raw walnuts or one tablespoon of flaxseed oil daily. If you use flaxseed oil, buy it fresh in a dark bottle, keep it refrigerated, use the oil within six weeks after opening, and don't heat it. Flaxseed oil is highly susceptible to deterioration when exposed to heat, light, or oxygen.

Gamma linolenic acid is an essential fatty acid that is not readily found in foods. Under ideal circumstances, the body makes GLA from fats and oils in the diet, but in reality, many factors interfere with the production of this important nutrient. The best and most reliable source of GLA is to take capsules of evening primrose, black currant, or borage seed oil. Take enough capsules so that you are obtaining between 120 and 240 mg of GLA daily.

Supplements for Overcoming Depression

Because low levels of many nutrients are associated with depression, it's helpful to take a high-potency vitamin and mineral supplement daily. The B-complex vitamins are particularly important in the treatment of mood disorders because they are critical for the production of neurotransmitters and a healthy nervous system.

Vitamin B6 helps to regulate mood, and is involved in the production of serotonin, a brain chemical that promotes feelings of well-being. People who are prone to depression tend to have low levels of both B6 and serotonin. Foods rich in B6 include whole grains, dark leafy greens, bananas, chicken, and avocados.

Vitamin B12 is also essential in the prevention and treatment of depression. This vitamin is found in animal proteins, but many people have deficiencies of vitamin B12 because it is not easily absorbed through the digestive tract. With age, the ability to absorb B12 becomes even weaker. If you suffer from depression, you may want to consider taking sublingual tablets of B12 in addition to a B-complex supplement. Sublingual tablets are dissolved under the tongue and absorbed directly into the bloodstream. Take one milligram of vitamin B12 every other day.

A lack of folic acid, another B vitamin, also causes depression and changes in personality. Folic acid occurs abundantly in leafy green vegetables, but because not many people eat sufficient amounts of leafy greens and the vitamin is destroyed by cooking, few people get sufficient amounts of this important vitamin. To ensure that you are getting adequate amounts these essential nutrients, buy a B-complex supplement that supplies 50–100 mg per day of B_1, B_2, B_3, B_5, and B_6, plus 400 mcg (micrograms) of folic acid.

Specific minerals also play a significant role in alleviating depression. Calcium and magnesium are two of the most important, and both help to calm the nervous system. Foods rich in calcium include dairy products, broccoli, kale, oranges, sesame seeds, sardines, and almonds. To ensure sufficient amounts of calcium, take 800–1,200 mg of supplemental calcium daily in the form of calcium citrate, which is the most easily absorbed form. For best assimilation, divide into two or three doses and take with meals.

Good dietary sources of magnesium include legumes, nuts, seeds, and whole grains. Again, to ensure sufficient levels of this necessary mineral, take 400–600 mg of supplemental magnesium daily in the form of citrate, malate, aspartate, gluconate, or lactate. Don't take more than 600 mg daily because excessive magnesium can cause diarrhea.

Diet and Lifestyle Stressors

Alcohol, tobacco, and caffeine all are contributing

factors to depression and are best avoided in the quest for improved mental and physical well-being. Alcohol is a significant depressant (that's why many people have a drink to relax). Although a drink or two several times a week may have some health benefits such as reducing cholesterol levels, if you are prone to depression, you are probably better off not drinking. Alcohol stimulates the production of adrenal hormones, which can increase feelings of anxiety. It also interferes with normal sleep cycles, and can contribute to insomnia. Drinking alcohol also causes blood sugar levels to drop, which contributes to hypoglycemia and mood swings.

Although caffeine is a socially acceptable beverage, it is a powerful and highly addictive drug. The stimulant effects of caffeine may be especially appealing to someone suffering from depression. Caffeine provides a momentary boost of energy and can help to clear thinking. However, people who are subject to anxiety or depression tend to be particularly susceptible to the effects of caffeine, and often experience nervousness, irritability, heart palpitations, and anxiety as a result. Several studies have found a direct correlation between coffee intake and depression. For some people, even the minute amount of caffeine found in decaffeinated coffee is enough to trigger anxiety and depressive symptoms.

Cigarette smoking is not generally considered as a factor in depressive disorders. However, nicotine stimulates the secretion of adrenal hormones,

Tryptophan
An essential amino acid that plays a role in the synthesis of serotonin.

including cortisol, the stress hormone. One of the effects of increased cortisol is to interfere with the amount of tryptophan that is delivered to the brain. Because serotonin levels are dependent upon tryptophan, serotonin is reduced.

At the same time, cortisol hinders serotonin receptors in the brain and makes them less responsive to the available serotonin.

Overcome Depression with Exercise

Exercise is one of the most powerful tools you have available for overcoming depression and keeping it at bay. In fact, regular daily exercise has been proven to be as effective as antidepressant drugs for relieving mild to moderate depression. In contrast to pharmaceutical drugs, the only side effects of exercise are beneficial and life-enhancing—exercise almost immediately changes your brain chemistry, and it provides a boost for your self-esteem.

Although all forms of exercise are helpful, aerobic exercise such as brisk walking, dancing, cross-country skiing, swimming, and bicycling appears to be the most beneficial for alleviating depression. Vigorous exercise stimulates the release of endorphins, the body's natural mood-elevating compounds.

Endorphins
Natural mood-elevating compounds produced naturally by the body in response to stimulus such as exercise.

In addition, aerobic exercise offers a healthy outlet for relieving feelings of irritability, frustration, and anger and encourages the shift to a more positive frame of mind. Studies have shown that people who exercise regularly not only have decreased symptoms of fatigue, anxiety, and depression, but they also have higher self-esteem than people who do not exercise. For the greatest benefit, exercise in the daylight. A moderate amount of sunlight improves mood by stimulating the production of mood-enhancing hormones and brain chemicals.

If you are depressed, you may feel lethargic and fatigued and not at all interested in exercising. But it's important to exercise even if you don't feel like it. Simply go out for a half-hour walk every day. If you are mildly depressed, you will probably feel your mood shift immediately. If you are suffering from more serious or chronic depression, it may take a few weeks of consistent exercise to notice a definite difference in your mood. Not only does exercise help to change your body chemistry to relieve depression, but establishing and following through with a regular program of exercise improves your self-confidence and enhances your ability to cope with the challenges that life presents.

The minimum amount of exercise that appears to be effective for preventing and relieving depression is approximately thirty minutes of activity five days a week. Early morning exercise seems to be most helpful for establishing a balanced and positive mood for the day, but exercise is beneficial at any time.

CHAPTER 9

A HOLISTIC APPROACH TO DEPRESSION

Approaching depression from a holistic standpoint involves considering the complex interaction of the body, mind, and spirit. Depressive disorders create ripples of pain that affect a human being on all levels—physical, mental, emotional, and spiritual. While medication can alleviate symptoms, no pill is a magic cure. From a holistic point of view, depression is an opportunity for self-empowerment and transformation.

The Deeper Meaning of Depression

The idea that depression may be a message from the soul has intrigued philosophers, poets, spiritual teachers, and psychotherapists for centuries. In our society, we idealize happiness, and busy ourselves with productivity to keep feelings at bay. There is little room for the sadness, emptiness, and loss that are also a part of normal life. But embracing these feelings and integrating them into our beings allows us to experience the full depth of our human nature, and contributes to our maturity.

Depression almost always carries a deeper message, and covering up or denying the feelings does not allow this deeper wisdom to rise to the surface of conscious awareness. Learning to tolerate feelings of sadness, grief, loneliness, anger, and the myriad of other emotions that we don't classify as "happy" can teach us much about ourselves.

This is not to say that you should live with debilitating depression. If you suffer from long-standing or severe depression, you should seek professional help. At the same time, begin to regard your depression as a messenger. Experiment with viewing melancholy as an opportunity for reflection. Take time to be quiet, to nurture yourself, and to ask your depression what it is trying to tell you.

Journaling for Self-Understanding

Depression is a signal that something is out of balance in your life. What is disturbing you? What feels overwhelming? What is dissatisfying about your life at this time? Writing down your feelings can be immensely helpful in this process of self-exploration. In fact, journaling on a regular basis has been shown in clinical studies to provide relief from depression and anxiety.

If you want to try journaling as a practice to ease depression, set aside approximately twenty minutes at a time when you can be alone. Write about your deepest thoughts and feelings, without consideration for grammar or spelling. Bypassing the intellect is essential for being able to access emotions. While you don't have to adhere to a schedule to benefit from journal writing, it does help to write frequently. Some people enjoy writing in the early morning, while others like to journal just before sleeping in order to process the day's events.

As scientists have pointed out, there does seem to be a definite link between disordered brain chemistry and depressive illness, but which comes first? The answer is most likely that sometimes, the depressed state comes first, which inhibits the production of feel-good brain chemicals. Other times, there is a genetic predisposition to low levels of mood-enhancing neurotransmitters, which can trigger depression. Either way, taking the time for self-reflection and giving your body, mind, and spirit the opportunity to come into a state of balance can only be beneficial and healing.

Meditation as a Path to Healing

Meditation is another helpful path to calming the mind and body. The regular practice of meditation helps you learn to observe the thoughts that pass through your mind, and to learn a healthy detachment from them that allows you to see the bigger picture. Meditation can help you recognize that your thoughts are simply thoughts—they are not you, they are not reality, they are simply the activity of your mind. In learning to meditate, you cultivate the ability to access a place of well-being in the midst of whatever may be going on in your life.

In addition, meditation helps in achieving an internal sense of balance and moderation, something that is sorely lacking in our society. Andrew Weil, M.D., is an advocate of meditation for alleviating depression. According to Weil, depression could just as easily be the result of disordered thinking causing biochemical brain changes—instead of current psychiatric theories, which maintain that disordered brain chemistry causes depression. He maintains that the result of constantly seeking the "highs" of life leads to depression because people then don't know how to live with the "lows" that necessarily follow. He suggests daily meditation as an alternative to constantly seeking stimulating experiences.

Focusing on your breath is an uncomplicated meditation practice. Your breath connects your mind and body, and when you consciously focus your attention on your breathing, you immediately and positively influence your physical and emotional well-being. By paying attention to your breathing and learning to consciously influence the rate and depth of your breath, you can significantly alter your emotional state.

To begin breathwork practice, find a quiet place where you will not be disturbed, and sit in a comfortable position. Bring your attention to your breathing. Relax, and inhale through your nose to a count of five, counting at a pace that is comfortable for you. Hold your breath for a count of five. Open your mouth slightly, and exhale to a count of ten, keeping your exhalation smooth and controlled. Repeat the exercise for a total of five complete cycles.

For a basic meditation practice, try focusing on a word or a phrase that you find calming and relaxing. You might try, "I am calm," or any other word or phrase that appeals to you. Sit or lie in a comfortable position, close your eyes, and take three slow, deep breaths, exhaling completely. Begin saying to yourself, "I am calm," with each exhalation. When your mind wanders, gently bring your attention back to your breathing and your calming phrase. Continue for twenty minutes, imagining waves of relaxation and well-being flowing throughout your body. The more you practice, the easier meditation becomes.

Focusing your complete awareness on a task such as bathing, cooking, or washing dishes is a way of bringing the principles of meditation into everyday life. To try this meditation practice, choose a routine task and focus your attention completely on what you are doing. Slow your movements down to about half of your normal pace. Pay close attention to your body, to each movement, and notice any feelings of tension or discomfort. Breathe into any tightness that you discover and consciously release the tension.

We often habitually perform daily tasks with much more effort than is needed. By paying close attention to your movements, you can learn to do whatever you need to do with the optimal expenditure of effort. This leaves your body relaxed and prevents the unnecessary buildup of stress and tension. This meditation practice is also a way of focusing your attention in the moment, and not allowing your mind to play the negative tapes that it is accustomed to running.

Psychotherapy and Depression

Psychotherapy, also known as "talk therapy," plays a central role in the successful treatment of a depressive disorder. In fact, in some cases of mild or even moderate depression, psychotherapy can be sufficient for alleviating depression. Many doctors still prescribe medication because of the quick symptom relief that can occur. But in most cases of depression, psychotherapy is necessary to address aspects of the illness that drugs do nothing to heal.

Drugs, including the natural alternative St. John's wort, can help to ease the physiological aspects of depressive disorders—the imbalance in brain chemistry that can make everyday functioning so difficult. But for long-term healing, people often need to learn more healthful ways of interacting with their environment. Healing the deep inner wounds that are often at the core of a depressive disorder generally requires intense inner work. A good therapist can help you understand and work through your feelings, and can also help you learn new ways of coping with life stressors that contribute to depression.

There are many different styles of psychotherapy. It's important to find a style of psychotherapy that works for you, and to find a therapist with whom you feel comfortable. Psychotherapy involves sharing your deepest thoughts and feelings, and you need to work with someone that you trust.

Although psychotherapists (including psychologists and clinical social workers) are highly trained professionals, they cannot prescribe medication. If you or your therapist believe that medication would be beneficial in the treatment of your depressive disorder, you must see your medical doctor or a psychiatrist for a prescription. If you are interested in trying St. John's wort, no prescription is necessary.

Cognitive therapy is one of the most successful of the psychotherapy approaches for alleviating depression. In cognitive therapy, the focus is on identifying and changing the thinking and behavior patterns that lead to depression. Depression is often related to low self-esteem and negative, self-defeating thoughts. In cognitive therapy, you learn to recognize and dispute the unconscious negative beliefs that permeate your thinking and to replace them with more realistic and self-affirming thoughts. It is often helpful to write down the thoughts as they occur, which helps in identifying and challenging the negative thoughts that run like cassette tapes through the subconscious mind. In cognitive therapy, you learn to change the way that you think about yourself.

One Step at a Time

Depression can be debilitating, both physically and emotionally. It's important to take steps to overcome depression, but at the same time, remember to be gentle with yourself and to set reasonable goals. Here are some things that can help.

Make a list each day of what you want to accomplish. Keep it simple and specific so that you don't end up feeling overwhelmed. Recall the activities that you enjoyed in the past, and make plans to engage in at least one activity each week, even if you don't feel like it. Schedule in at least thirty minutes of aerobic exercise every day—even a brisk walk is sufficient. Spend time with people that you like, and share your feelings with someone that you trust.

Don't expect your mood to change immediately, but cultivate awareness of small improvements in how you feel and the ways that you engage in life. You may find it encouraging to make a list at the end of each day, noting the positive steps you took during the day to help yourself feel better.

Take Time to Nurture Yourself

Time for self-nurturing is often last on the list of things to do in our overly busy, productivity-obsessed society. But without some regular time out from the activities of daily life, it's easy to become exhausted physically, mentally, and spiritually. With the challenges of juggling family, career, home, and social responsibilities, it's even more essential to set aside time for yourself to indulge in the activities that you find restorative for your body, mind, and soul. Neglecting this important aspect of self-care sets the stage for the emptiness and fatigue that we label as depression.

Make self-nurturing a priority, and you will most likely find that you have more energy and enthusiasm for engaging in daily life. Begin by making a list of your favorite ways of caring for yourself, the things that bring you pleasure and make you feel glad to be alive. Include things for your body (receiving a massage, soaking in an aromatherapy bath, talking a walk in nature); for your mind (reading a new book, going to a lecture that interests you, watching a favorite movie); and for your soul (listening to sacred music, talking intimately with a friend, visiting an art gallery).

Each week, set aside time for engaging in at least one activity for each aspect of your being—

one thing to nurture your body, one for your mind, and one for your soul. Schedule your appointments for self-nurturing on your calendar, just as you would any other important engagement.

Establish Community

People who are depressed often report a sense of isolation and loneliness. The sense of separation from others that characterizes our modern society is a recent phenomenon. Human beings naturally gravitate toward living in community, and when deprived of close contact, begin to feel disconnected and alone. Even if your family of origin is not made up of people that you would choose as close friends, you can still create a sense of family and intimacy in your life.

Building a network of loving support and friendship takes time and effort, and you might find it difficult to reach out if you're feeling depressed. Start slowly, but make it a goal to do one thing each day to connect with someone that you think you might like to know better. Invite a neighbor over for tea; attend a lecture or meeting on something that interests you and stay around afterward to socialize; join a group or service organization; attend a church, synagogue, or other religious service; join a health club, exercise class, or yoga class; volunteer for a cause you believe in. Make it a goal to have at least a half-dozen people in your life with whom you can share your deepest thoughts and feelings, and with whom you enjoy spending time.

CHAPTER 10

SAFETY AND
PRECAUTIONS

Because St. John's wort is marketed as a nutritional supplement and not as a drug, it does
not fall under the regulation of the Food and Drug
Administration (this is true for all herbal supplements). To further complicate the issue, most con-
ventionally trained doctors do not receive training
in botanical medicine. This means that your doctor
may not be fully aware of the beneficial properties
of St. John's wort and may not know exactly how to
prescribe it, or what cautions should be observed.

Herbs Are Powerful Medicines

Many people have the erroneous belief that because a substance is derived from a plant, it cannot
be harmful. Herbs have healing benefits because
they contain compounds that have measurable biological effects on the body. Some of these compounds are potentially harmful if the plant is used
improperly.

The renaissance of interest in herbal medicine
in this country indicates that the general public is
tired of the side effects and costs of prescription
medications, and that people are interested in a
more natural, less invasive approach to healing.
Herbal remedies also offer the opportunity for a
more empowered role of health care, one that en-
ables individuals to assume a more active role in
their healing. This freedom also means that it is es-

sential to be educated about the substances that you take into your body, whether these substances are prescription drugs or herbs.

Possible Side Effects of St. John's Wort

The long history of safety of St. John's wort makes it a valuable alternative to prescription antidepressants for many people. Most people can use St. John's wort safely, but as with any medicinal herb or drug, certain precautions should be observed. If you are taking St. John's wort, be sure to tell your doctor, because the herb may affect other medications that you are taking. Do not take St. John's wort if you are pregnant without consulting your doctor.

Side effects occasionally occur with St. John's wort, but they tend to be minor and uncommon. Some people report mild stomach upset while taking the herb. Taking St. John's wort with food can help to prevent digestive upset. More rarely, some people experience allergic reactions, fatigue, or restlessness while using St. John's wort. If you notice any of these symptoms, consult your health care practitioner for advice before continuing to use the herb.

At one time, St. John's wort was thought to act in a similar way to monoamine oxidase inhibitors (MAOIs), an older class of antidepressant drugs. For this reason, people taking St. John's wort were cautioned to avoid foods high in the amino acid tyramine (such as red wine, aged cheese, and chocolate) because the interaction of these foods with MAO inhibitors can cause blood pressure levels to become dangerously elevated. Symptoms of this reaction include headaches, palpitations, and nausea. But more recent research has not confirmed that St. John's wort is an MAO inhibitor. Instead, St. John's wort is thought to act more like the more recent class of antidepressant drugs that increase levels of serotonin in the brain.

St. John's Wort and Photosensitivity

St. John's wort is classified as toxic to livestock because it can cause severe photosensivity (adverse reaction to sunlight). Although this reaction is uncommon in humans, there have been a few reports of photosensivity in people taking therapeutic amounts of St. John's wort.

Symptoms of photosensitivity include skin rash, unusual susceptibility to sunburn, or pain or burning of the skin when exposed to ultraviolet light. Fair-skinned people are most vulnerable, as are people who have experienced reactions to ultraviolet light when taking other types of medications. If you are at risk for photosensitivity, take care to avoid excessive sun exposure, tanning lamps, or other sources of ultraviolet light while taking St. John's wort.

The Effect of St. John's Wort on Prescription Drugs

Research reported by the National Institutes of Health in early 2000 revealed that St. John's wort may reduce the effectiveness of some prescription drugs. As a result, the Food and Drug Administration asked health care professionals to caution patients about the potential risks of combining St. John's wort with other medications. However, this does not mean that St. John's wort can never be used in combination with prescription drugs. It simply means that to be safe, you should always let your doctor know about any herbal supplements that you may be using to avoid the possibility of harmful drug interactions.

St. John's wort appears to speed up metabolic activity in a key pathway that is responsible for the breakdown of some prescription drugs. Basically, this means that the body processes the drugs more quickly, which lowers blood levels of the medications and decreases the effectiveness of the drugs.

Specifically, St. John's wort has been found to affect indinavir and other protease inhibitors, which are antiviral drugs used to treat HIV infection. St. John's wort also apparently affects cyclosporin, which is used to help prevent organ rejection in patients who have undergone transplants. In addition, St. John's wort may affect other immunosuppressant drugs and other medications that work through the same pathway. This includes birth control pills, cholesterol-lowering medications such as Mevacor (lovastatin), other drugs used in heart disease such as digoxin, some cancer medications, seizure drugs, and blood thinners such as Coumadin (warfarin). If you are taking these drugs, taking St. John's wort may interfere with their effectiveness and could potentially cause dangerous changes in drug effects. To be safe, always inform your doctor about any herbs and supplements that you are taking.

St. John's Wort and Antidepressants

If you are currently taking antidepressant medications, it is essential that you work with your doctor if you are interested in taking St. John's wort. Do not attempt to abruptly discontinue antidepressants, but instead, work with your doctor to gradually wean yourself from prescription medications. Also, be aware that in some cases (especially for people with major chronic depression and those with bipolar disorder) prescription medications are probably necessary. Hyla Cass, M.D., offers a protocol helpful for physicians and patients for substituting St. John's wort for antidepressants in her book *St. John's Wort: Nature's Blues Buster.*

CHAPTER 11

HOW TO BUY AND USE ST. JOHN'S WORT

St. John's wort is a top-selling herb and is widely available in natural food stores and pharmacies. Choosing among the dozens of St. John's wort products can be confusing. In this chapter, you will learn how to identify good-quality products and understand the differences among the various herbal formulations. With this information, you will be able to make an informed decision that will help you choose a product that best meets your needs. You will also learn how to take St. John's wort and the dosages that are most effective.

Please note that if you are suffering from anything other than very mild depression, you should be working with a health professional who can provide you with appropriate support and guidance.

Finding an Effective Supplement

There can be a vast difference in the way that St. John's wort is grown, harvested, and processed. As a result, there can be significant differences in the quality of commercial St. John's wort products. While some products are good sources of the beneficial compounds that make St. John's wort so effective, others may contain little or none of the active ingredients. While all parts of the plant contain some degree of plant chemicals, the flower buds of St. John's wort contain the highest concentrations of the active ingredients.

In 1998, the *Los Angeles Times* commissioned laboratory tests on ten different St. John's wort products. The researchers found that the potencies of the products were very different from what was claimed on the label. Because manufacturers want consumers to have confidence in the herbal products they are buying, the herbal industry is moving toward third-party certification, such as is provided by the U.S. Pharmocopeia, a nonprofit group that establishes drug standards, and NSF International, a nonprofit group that sets health standards. This means that herbal products are tested by an independent group to ensure that the products meet certain standards. In the process, the consumer is assured of a quality product.

Different Forms of St. John's Wort

St. John's wort is available in many different forms, including as teas, capsules, tablets, and liquid extracts. You'll even find St. John's wort included in some foods, such as breakfast cereals and snacks. The addition of St. John's wort to food products is a marketing strategy that capitalizes on the popularity of St. John's wort, and is not meant for the treatment of depressive disorders.

St. John's wort has traditionally been used as a tea and as a tincture (a liquid extract made by crushing and steeping the herb in food-grade alcohol). Teas made from St. John's wort are not recommended for treating depression, because the active ingredients are not adequately extracted in hot water. Tinctures (now labeled as liquid extracts by manufacturers) do extract the active chemicals. Of course, this depends on the initial quality of the plant material and the care of the manufacturer during the processing of the plant.

The amount of active ingredients can vary greatly in liquid extracts. If you want to try taking a liquid extract, the Herb Research Foundation suggests taking 20 to 30 drops three times a day. Dilute the extract with a small amount of warm water or add to juice, and take it with meals.

Standardized Extracts

All of the research on St. John's wort has been conducted using standardized extracts, which makes it easier for researchers to maintain consistency in their studies. While St. John's wort products do not have to be standardized to be effective, if you want to be sure that you are obtaining adequate levels of the active compounds, your best bet is to buy products that are labeled as standardized extracts.

Standardized extracts are herbal products that are guaranteed to contain a specified amount of what is currently believed to be the herb's primary active ingredient. Various processes are used to obtain the specified concentration, including removing what are considered to be unimportant constituents and adding high concentrations of the isolated active ingredients.

St. John's wort extracts are typically standardized to contain 0.3 percent hypericin and 5 percent hyperforin. If you are using a standardized extract, buy products that state on the label that they contain these percentages of active ingredients.

Standardization
Standardized extracts are herbal products guaranteed to contain a specified amount of the herb's primary active ingredients.

Although most of the research on St. John's wort has used 900 mg daily of St. John's wort (usually taken as 300 mg three times a day), people vary in their response to the herb and you can adjust the dosage as needed. Some people respond well to lesser amounts of the herb, while others need more.

It's safe to take as much as 1,800 mg of St.

John's wort daily, but you should give the herb at least two months at the standard amount of 900 mg before increasing your dosage. To increase the amount you are taking, add an additional 300 mg daily for one month, and then continue adding an additional 300 mg daily dosage each month until you reach 1,800 mg. Working with a health practitioner who is familiar with St. John's wort can be helpful in determining the dosage that is most appropriate for you.

It's best to take the full amount of the herb in three equal doses, one with each meal. Taking the herb with a meal helps to prevent the possibility of any digestive upset. Taking St. John's wort at regular intervals throughout the day keeps a steady supply of the active ingredients available to your body. Many people notice a significant difference within a couple of weeks of taking St. John's wort, and report improvements in sleep quality, energy levels, and appetite. But don't be discouraged if you don't notice changes right away. It can take several weeks for the full effects of St. John's wort to kick in.

Seeing Results from St. John's Wort

The most common mistake that people make when taking herbal supplements is in not giving the herb sufficient time to have a physiological effect on the body. You should expect definite results, but be patient and give the herb at least six weeks before making a decision about whether or not to continue taking it.

It's important to take the herb regularly, not just when you're feeling depressed. St. John's wort has a cumulative positive effect on depression, and interrupting your regular schedule of taking the herb can diminish the benefits. However, don't fret if you happen to miss a dosage. Just try to keep as much as possible to a regular schedule of taking the herb. If necessary, you can always double up on a dosage if you happen to miss one.

If you're not getting positive results from St. John's wort within six to eight weeks, it's possible that the supplement you are taking may not contain adequate amounts of the active compounds to be effective. For this reason, it is essential to buy quality herbal products from a reputable company. Ask your doctor, pharmacist, or a qualified herbalist for recommendations.

How Long to Take St. John's Wort

As your depression lifts and your mood stabilizes, you may want to consider beginning to taper off of St. John's wort. For most people, staying on the herb for at least one month after depressive symptoms have abated is helpful. Although there are generally no negative side effects associated with discontinuing St. John's wort, you may want to taper off of it gradually, lessening your dosage by 300 mg at a time over a period of weeks. While many people do take St. John's wort for brief periods, others find that they do best when they take the herb for months, or even years. St. John's wort can be taken for as long as is necessary and can be used safely for an indefinite period of time.

Because it can be difficult to self-evaluate progress in depressive disorders, you may find it useful to retake the depression test in this book once a month while you are using St. John's wort, and also during the time when you are decreasing your dosage of the herb. It's also best to work with a mental health professional who can guide you in your treatment plan.

Depressive disorders are complex, and the successful path to a satisfying way of life requires a commitment to healing on all levels. Combined with attention to your physical, emotional, and spiritual well-being, St. John's wort can be a valuable ally in your journey.

SELECTED REFERENCES

American Herbal Pharmacopoeia and Therapeutic Compendium. "St. John's Wort (*Hypericum Performatum*) Monograph." *Herbalgram: The Journal of the American Botanical Council and the Herb Research Foundation,* 1997; 40:1–16.

Barnes J, Anderson LA, Phillipson JD. "St. John's wort (Hypericum perforatum L.): a review of its chemistry, pharmacology and clinical properties." *Journal Pharm Pharmacol,* 2001; 53:583–600.

Brenner R, Azbel V, Madhusoodanan S, Pawlowska M. "Comparison of an extract of hypericum (LI 160) and sertraline in the treatment of depression: a double-blind, randomized pilot study." *Clin Ther,* 2000; 22:411–418.

Grube B, Walper A, Wheatley D. "St. John's wort extract: efficacy for menopausal symptoms of psychological origin." *Adv Ther,* 1999; 16:177–186.

Huebner WD, Kirste T. "Experience with St. John's wort (*Hypericum performatum*) in children under 12 years with symptoms of depression and psychovegetative disturbances." *Phytotherapy Research* 2001; 15:367–370.

Kalb R, Troutman-Sponsel RD, Kieser M. "Efficacy and tolerability of Hypericum extract WS 5572 versus placebo in mildly to moderately depressed patients." *Pharmacopsychiatry,* 2001; 34: 96–103.

Linde K, Ramirez G, Mulrow CD, Weidenhammer W, and Melchart D. "St. John's wort for depression—an overview and metaanalysis of randomized clinical trials." *British Medical Journal*, 1996; 313:253–258.

Philipp M, Kohnen R, Hiller KO. "Hypericum extract versus imipramine or placebo in patients with moderate depression: randomised multicentre study of treatment for eight weeks." *British Medical Journal*, 1999; 319:1534–1538.

Schrader E. "Equivalence of St. John's wort extract (Ze 117) and fluoxetine: a randomized, controlled study in mild-moderate depression." *Int Clin Psychopharmacol*, 2000; 15:61–68.

Stevinson C, Ernst E. "A pilot study of Hypericum perforatum for the treatment of premenstrual syndrome." *BJOG*, 2000; 107:870–876.

Woelk H. "Comparison of St. John's wort and imipramine for treating depression: randomised controlled trial." *British Medical Journal*, 2000; 321:536–539.

OTHER BOOKS
AND RESOURCES

Burns, D. *Feeling Good: The New Mood Therapy*. New York, NY: Whole Care Publishing, 1999.

Cass, H. *St. John's Wort: Nature's Blues Buster*. Garden City Park, NY: Avery Publishing Group, 1998.

Glenmullen, J. *Prozac Backlash: Overcoming the Dangers of Prozac, Zoloft, Paxil, and Other Antidepressants with Safe, Effective Alternatives*. New York, NY: Simon and Schuster, 2000.

Murray, M. and Pizzorno, J. *Encyclopedia of Natural Medicine*. Rocklin, CA: Prima Publishing, 1998.

Vukovic, L. *Herbal Healing Secrets for Women*. Paramus, NJ: Prentice Hall, 2000.

Vukovic, L. *Journal of Desires: A Daily Diary with Readings and Reflections Guiding You to Fulfillment of Your Lifelong Wishes and Dreams*. Paramus, NJ: Prentice Hall, 2001.

GreatLife Magazine
Consumer magazine with articles on vitamins, minerals, herbs, and foods.
Available for free at many health and natural food stores.

Let's Live Magazine
Consumer magazine with emphasis on the health benefits of vitamins, minerals, and herbs.

Customer service:
1-800-676-4333
P.O. Box 74908
Los Angeles, CA 90004

Subscriptions: 12 issues per year, $19.95 in the U.S.; $31.95 outside the U.S.

Physical Magazine
Magazine oriented to body builders and other serious athletes.

Customer service:
1-800-676-4333
P.O. Box 74908
Los Angeles, CA 90004

Subscriptions: 12 issues per year, $19.95 in the U.S.; $31.95 outside the U.S.

The Nutrition Reporter™ newsletter
Monthly newsletter that summarizes recent medical research on vitamins, minerals, and herbs.

Customer service:
P.O. Box 30246
Tucson, AZ 85751-0246
e-mail: jack@thenutritionreporter.com
www.nutritionreporter.com

Subscriptions: $26 per year (12 issues) in the U.S.; $32 U.S. or $48 CNC for Canada; $38 for other countries

National Institute of Mental Health
Information Resources and Inquiries Branch
6001 Executive Boulevard
Bethesda, MD 20892-9663
1-800-421-4211
http://www.nimh.nih.gov

National Depressive and Manic Depressive Association

730 N. Franklin Street, Suite 501
Chicago, IL 60610
1-800-82-NDMA
http://www.ndmda.org

INDEX

Printed in the USA
CPSIA information can be obtained
at www.ICGtesting.com
JSHW012009140824
68134JS00004B/89